THE
WELLBEING
JOURNAL

THE
WELLBEING
JOURNAL

Creative Activities
to Inspire

In aid of

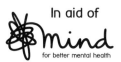
for better mental health

All royalties from the sale of this book (a minimum of
£5,000) will be donated to Mind, a registered charity
in England and Wales (charity number 219830).

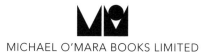

MICHAEL O'MARA BOOKS LIMITED

First published in Great Britain in 2017
by Michael O'Mara Books Limited
9 Lion Yard
Tremadoc Road
London SW4 7NQ

A CIP catalogue record for this book is available from the British Library.

Papers used by Michael O'Mara Books Limited are natural, recyclable
products made from wood grown in sustainable forests. The manufacturing
processes conform to the environmental regulations of the country of origin.

ISBN: 978-1-78243-800-7 in paperback print format

16

www.mombooks.com

Designed by Claire Cater
Illustrated by Kirsten Sevig

Every reasonable effort has been made to acknowledge all copyright holders.
Any errors or omissions that may have occurred are inadvertent, and anyone
with any copyright queries is invited to write to the publisher, so that full
acknowledgement may be included in subsequent editions of the work.

Printed and bound in China

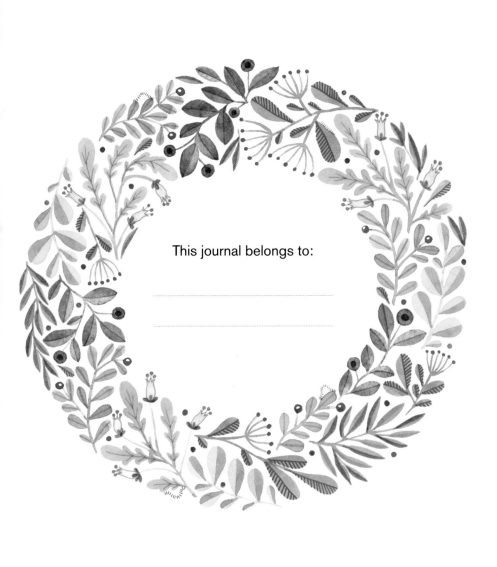

This journal belongs to:

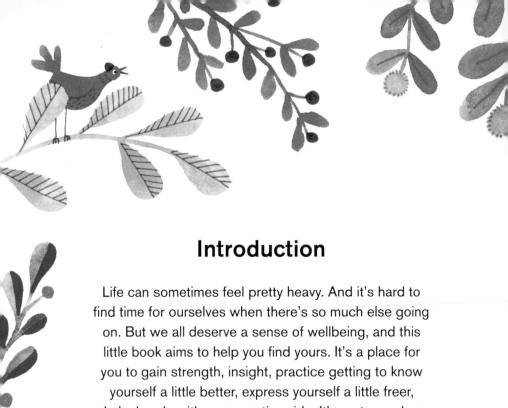

Introduction

Life can sometimes feel pretty heavy. And it's hard to find time for ourselves when there's so much else going on. But we all deserve a sense of wellbeing, and this little book aims to help you find yours. It's a place for you to gain strength, insight, practice getting to know yourself a little better, express yourself a little freer, shake hands with your creative side. It's up to you how to use it – diary, sketchpad, list-keeper, coaster – but whatever you do, we hope you enjoy it.
And we hope it helps.

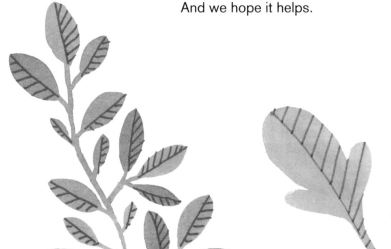

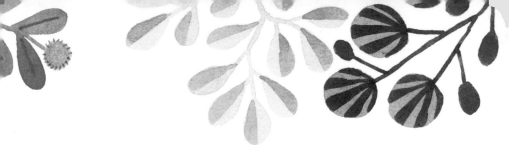

The Wellbeing Journal is published by Michael O'Mara Books, to raise money and awareness for Mind, the mental health charity. All royalties from the sale of this book (a minimum of £5,000) will be donated to Mind, a registered charity in England and Wales (charity number 219830).

Mind believes that no one should have to face a mental health problem alone. We're here for you. Today. Now. We're on your doorstep, on the end of a phone or online. Whether you're stressed, depressed or in crisis. We'll listen, give you support and advice, and fight your corner.

If you need us:
Mind Infoline: 0300 123 3393
or text: 86463
9am to 6pm, Monday to Friday (except for bank holidays)

info@mind.org.uk
Find your local Mind at mind.org.uk/localmind

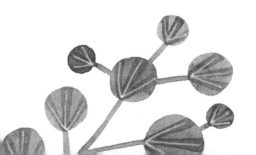
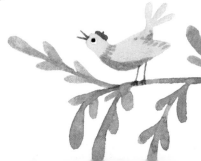

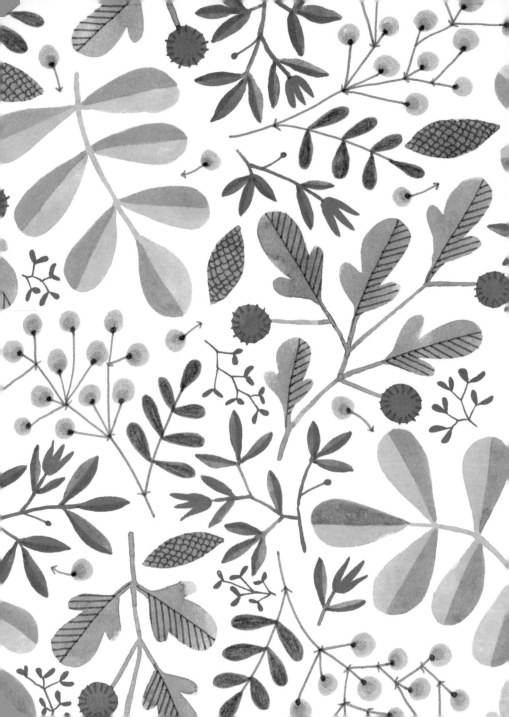

A Spot of Colouring

Colouring is a simple and relaxing way of taking time
for yourself. It can be a helpful practice if you find
it hard to switch off as it allows the mind to slow
down and become absorbed without strain.

Try it for yourself with the pattern opposite. Take your
time selecting the colours you want to use. Then spend
a minute or two looking at the intricacies in the pattern
before you start. When you're ready, begin to colour.

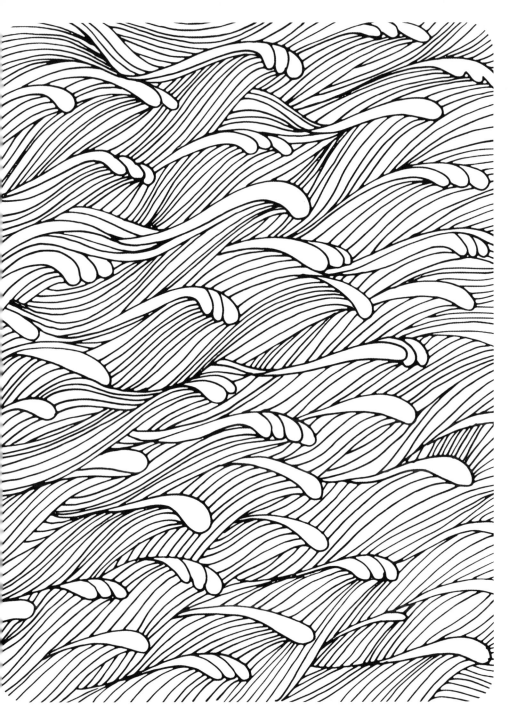

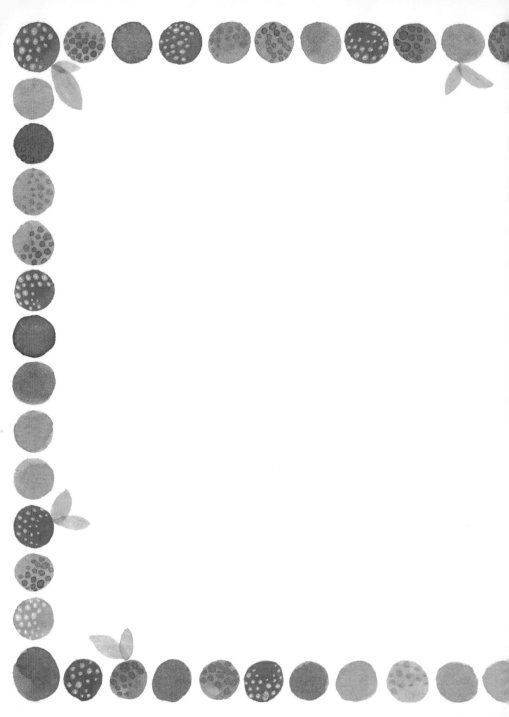

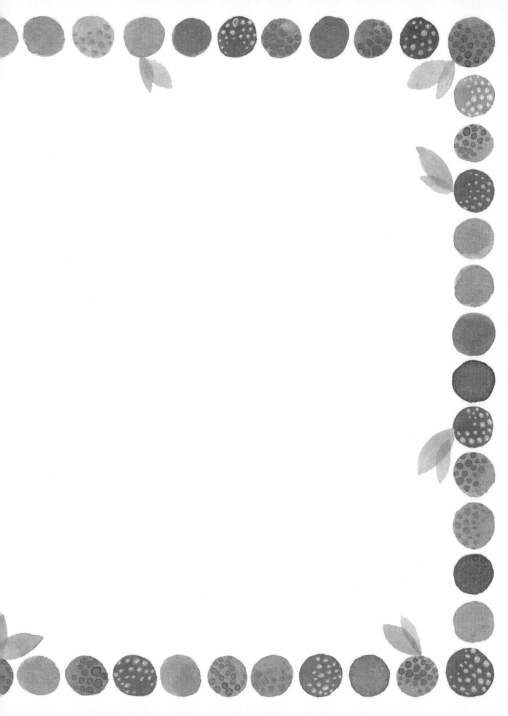

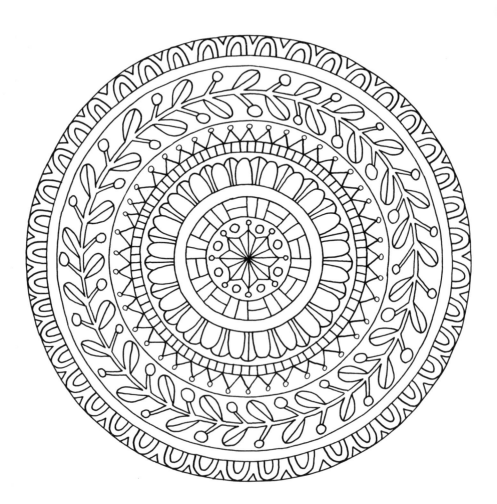

'Adopt the pace of
nature: her secret
is patience.'

Ralph Waldo Emerson

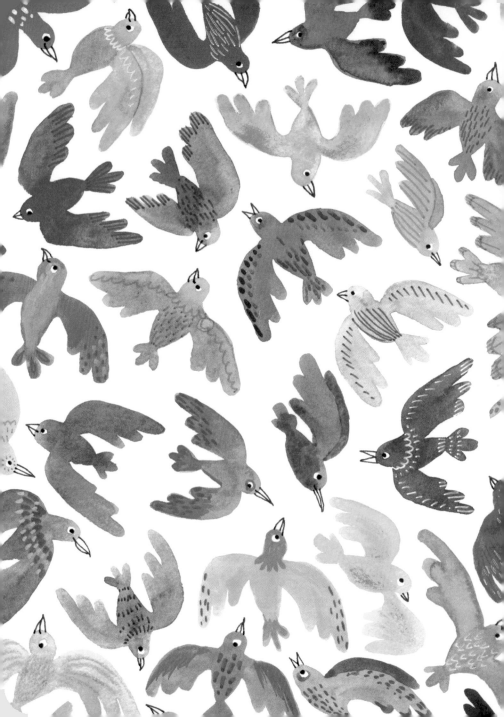

Relax Your Body

When you're stressed, your muscles can become
tight and tense. This exercise helps you notice
tension in your body and relax your muscles.

Lie down or sit with your back straight and your feet on the
floor. Close your eyes or focus on a spot in the distance.

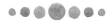

Start by clenching your toes as much as you can
for a few seconds then releasing them. Notice
the difference between the two feelings.

Match this to your breathing. Tense each muscle as you
take a deep breath in, and relax as you breathe out.

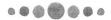

Move up your body to your thighs, your stomach and all the way
to your shoulders and hands, clenching and relaxing each muscle
in turn. Take time to notice any parts of your body that feel tense,
tight or tired. You can repeat these steps if you still feel tense.

Take a moment to relax, then slowly and gently begin to
move. When you feel ready you can stand up slowly.

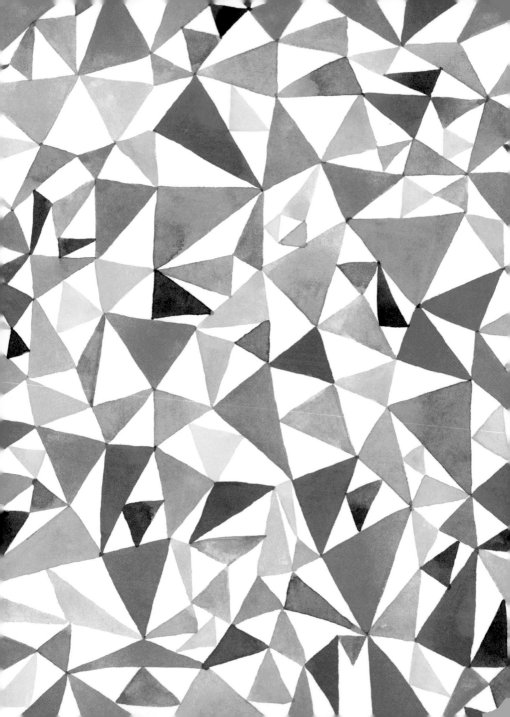

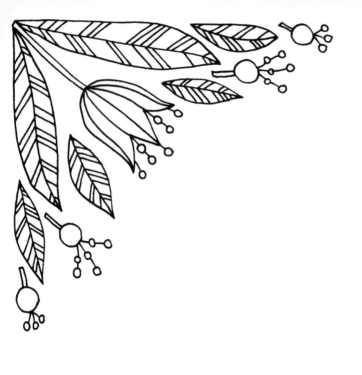
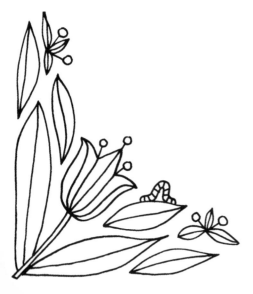

Get Creative

Doing something creative can help you feel
more calm and relaxed. It works by:

distracting you from worrying thoughts

giving you an outlet and focus for your emotions

stimulating your senses

You could try painting, drawing, making crafts, playing a musical
instrument, dancing, baking or sewing. The key is to try not to worry
too much about the finished product, and focus on enjoying yourself.

Even a few minutes spent doing something creative can
make a difference. Try using the shapes and patterns
opposite to get started with a bit of doodling.

'I found I could say
things with colour
and shapes that I
couldn't say any
other way.'

Georgia O'Keeffe

What Do You Enjoy?

Life can be hectic, and many of us don't feel that we have
time to fit in the things we enjoy. We focus our energy
on what we have to do and not what we want to do.
And when we have a little time for ourselves, we don't
tend to give it the attention or respect it deserves.

What do you enjoy doing? Perhaps it's seeing friends, cooking
a meal or sitting down with a book. It might be getting into
the outdoors on a walk or something more adventurous.

Take some time now to really consider what
makes you feel good and write a list here. Then
plan for when you're next going to do it.

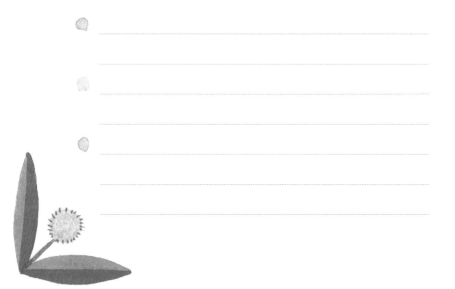

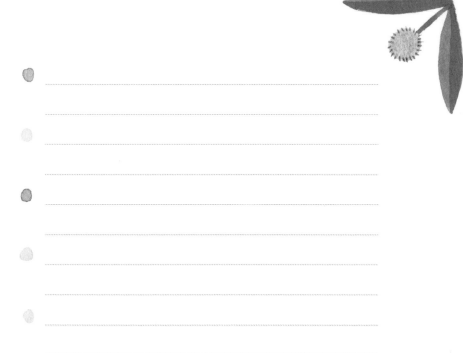

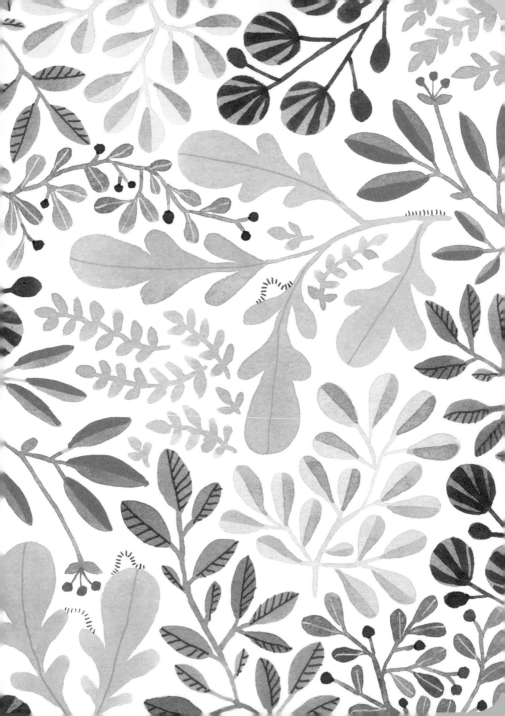

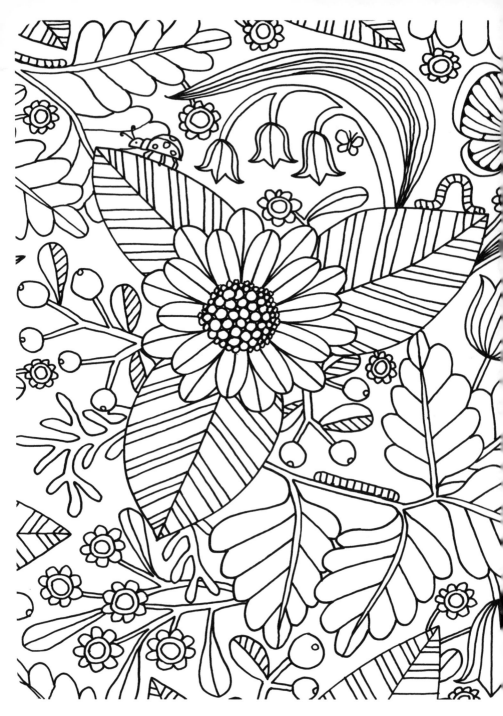

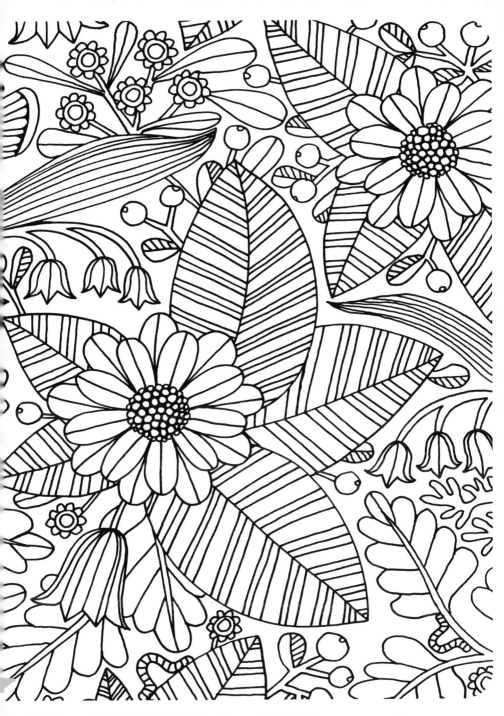

How Are You?

How do you feel right now? Can you describe it? Does
it have a colour? A shape? Can you draw it?

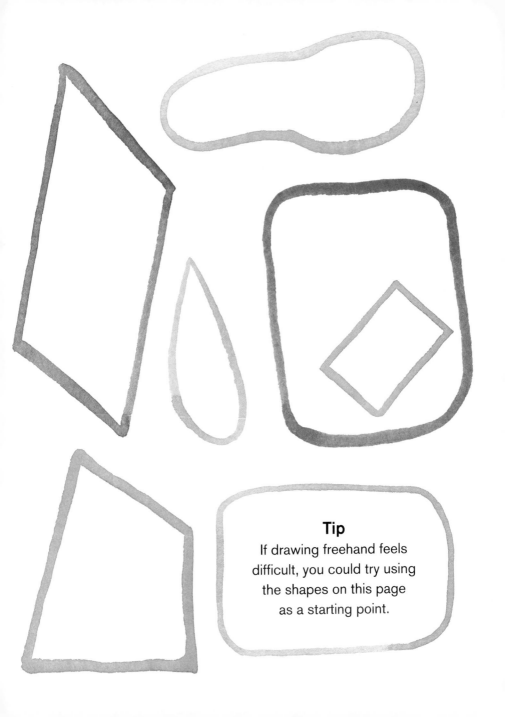

Tip
If drawing freehand feels
difficult, you could try using
the shapes on this page
as a starting point.

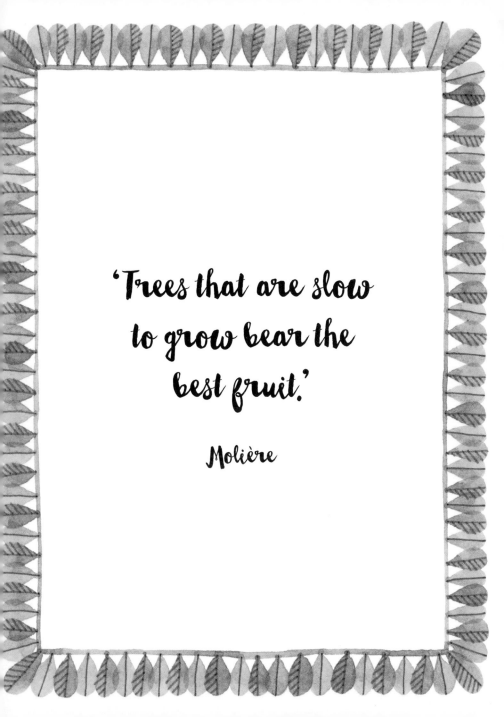

'Trees that are slow
to grow bear the
best fruit.'

Molière

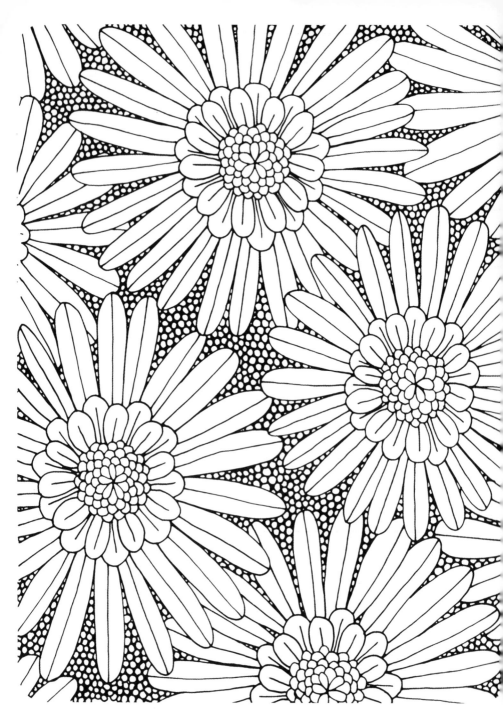

Take a Break

When you're feeling tense, taking just a short break can
have a surprising impact, bringing stress levels down
and making you more able to tackle the tasks ahead.

Try to give your break a focus (a relaxed focus, of course),
to take your mind away from any worries. A short walk
can be enough, or you could try listening to your favourite
songs. Turn up the volume and dance or sing along, or
put your headphones on and close your eyes. Really listen
to the music. Can you pick out different instruments?
Can you hear a drumbeat or a particular rhythm? Focus
on the music, and let other thoughts fade away.

Alternatively, if you haven't got much time, you could
sit down and colour in part of the pattern opposite.

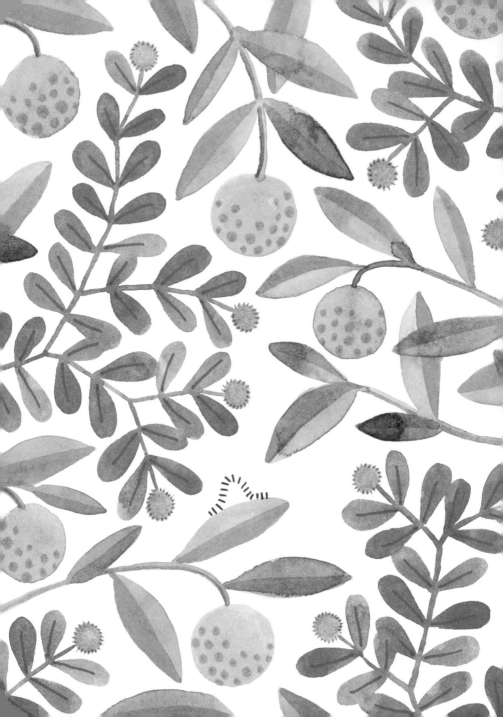

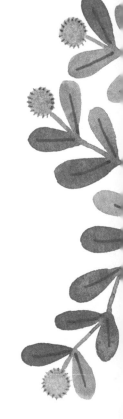
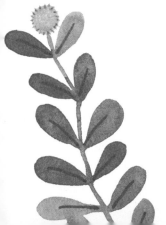

Organize Your Time

Making some adjustments to the way you organize your time can be a simple way of helping you to feel more in control of any tasks you're facing and more able to handle pressure.

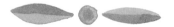

Identify your best time of day – you might be a morning person or an evening person – and do the important tasks that need the most energy and concentration at that time.

Make a list of things you have to do. Arrange them in order of importance and try to focus on the most urgent first. If your tasks are work related, ask a manager or colleague to help you prioritize. You may be able to push back some tasks until you're feeling more able to do them.

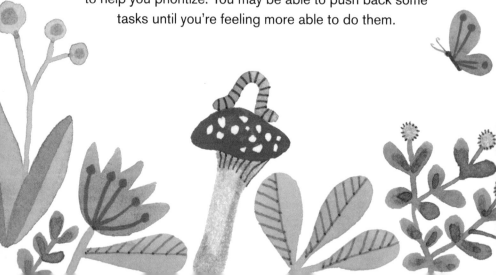

Vary your activities. Balance interesting tasks with more mundane ones, and difficult tasks with those you find easier or can do more calmly.

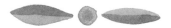

Try not to do too much at once. It sounds obvious but we all do it. Multitasking can not only make it harder for you to carry out any individual task well, it can also increase the sense of pressure.

Take breaks and avoid rushing. It might be difficult to do this when you're stressed, but it can make you more productive.

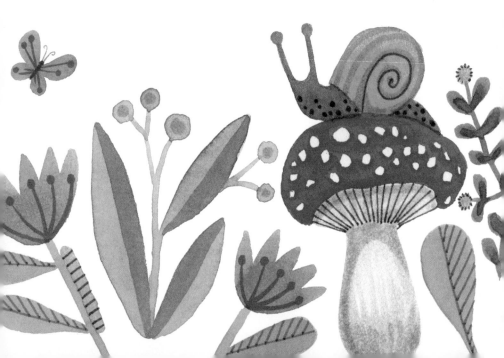

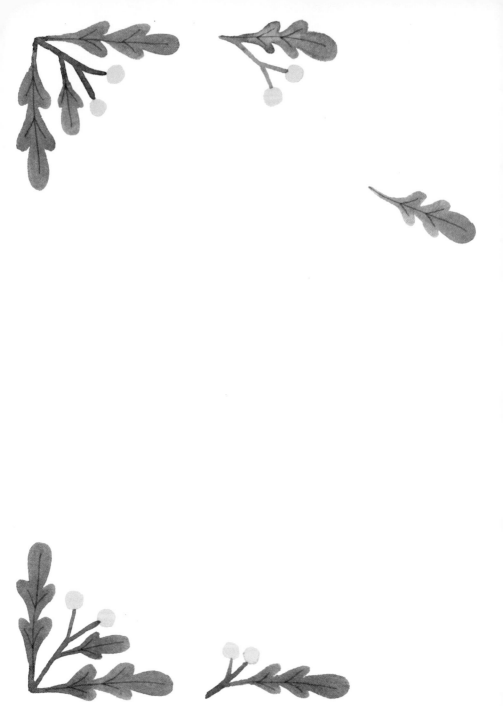

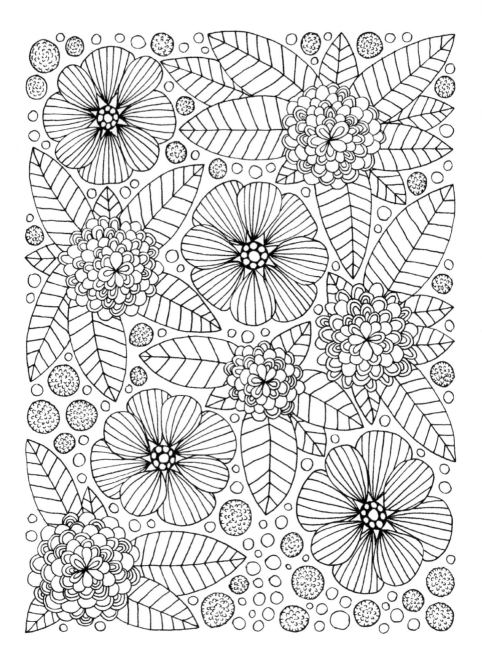

'In the midst of winter, I found there was, within me, an invincible summer.'

Albert Camus

Thoughts and Feelings

Each day this week fill in one of these squares with a picture of how you're feeling – turn back to 'How Are You?' for some tips on how to get started. At the end of the week look back at your record and spend some time thinking about how your feelings changed.

If you find this exercise helpful, you could use a blank calendar or diary to keep a longer record.

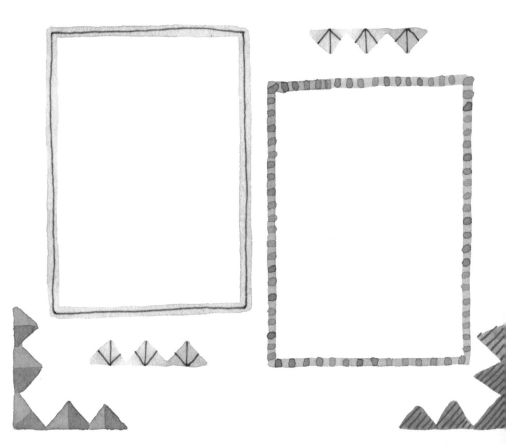

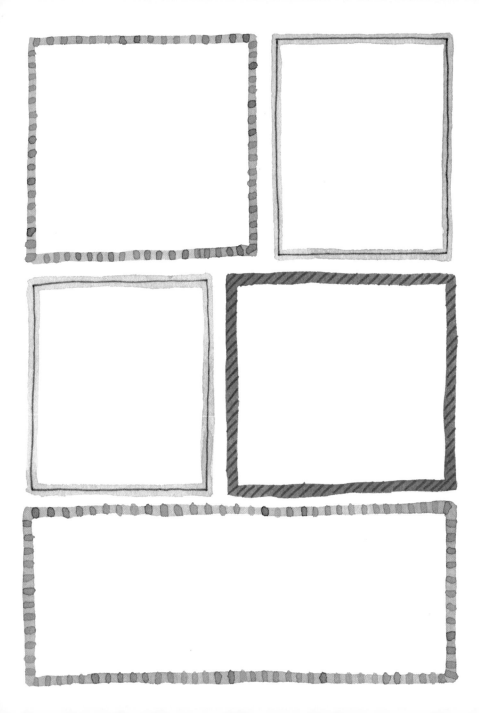

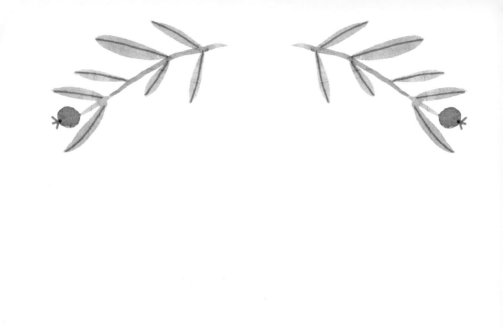

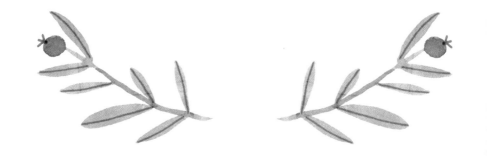

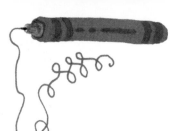

Pen to Paper

The next time you need to relax try
this simple drawing exercise.

1. Make sure you are sitting comfortably with your feet firmly on the floor, your back straight and your shoulders relaxed.

2. Take your pen, and draw a circle that fills most of the page – don't worry if it's a bit wonky!

3. Now keep drawing. You could keep going over the circle or fill it with a pattern, but try not to let your pen leave the page. Don't worry about creating a finished picture, just keep going.

4. Take time to focus on what you're drawing.

5. While you're drawing consider how the pen feels on the page, the sound it makes, how the colour comes out when you draw fast and when you draw slow.

6. Focusing on these sensations can help you quieten your mind, like meditation.

7. Once you have done this for a few minutes, try using a different colour or pattern.

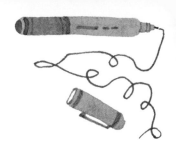

Tips

If you're focusing too much
on getting the pattern right,
try using your other hand.

•

If you find it hard to get started, it
can sometimes help to begin with
some colouring, just to loosen up.

'Creativity is contagious. Pass it on.'

Albert Einstein

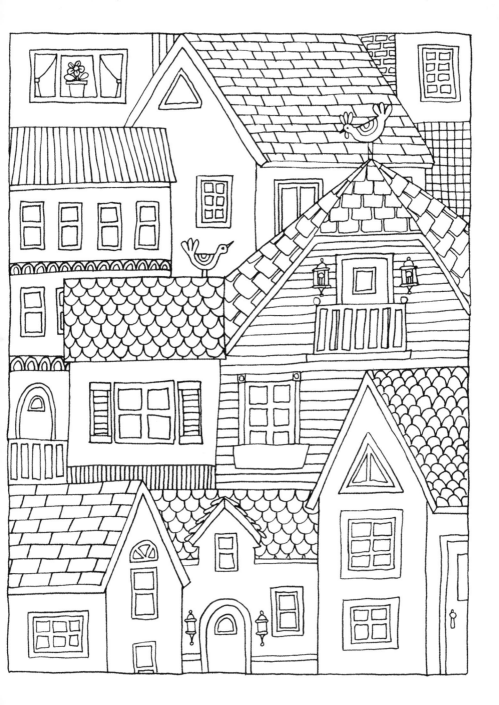

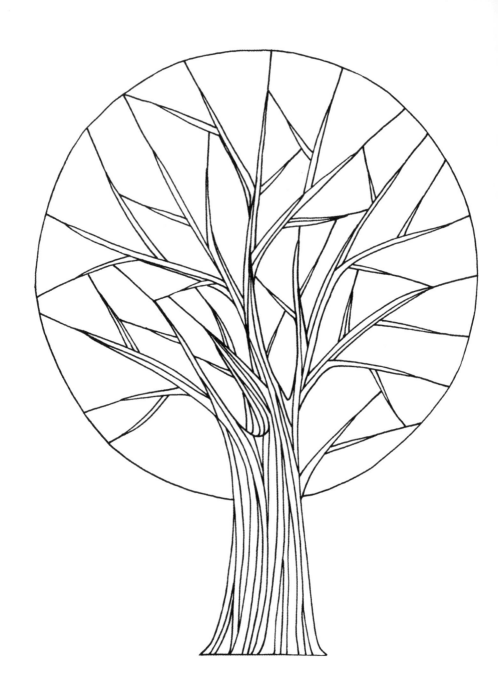

The Power of Green

Spending time outside and in green spaces can be great for your physical and mental wellbeing. To get the benefits you could:

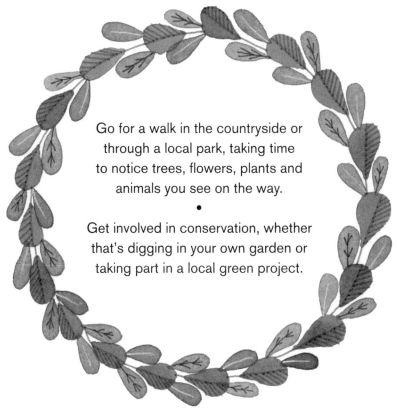

Go for a walk in the countryside or through a local park, taking time to notice trees, flowers, plants and animals you see on the way.

•

Get involved in conservation, whether that's digging in your own garden or taking part in a local green project.

If you don't have time to go out into nature now, bring some of the power of green things inside by colouring the page opposite using different shades of green. If you've only got one green pen or pencil you could fill the segments with different patterns, such as stripes or spots or cross-hatching.

'The earth has its music for those who will listen.'

Reginald Vincent Holmes

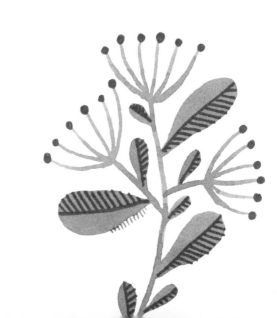

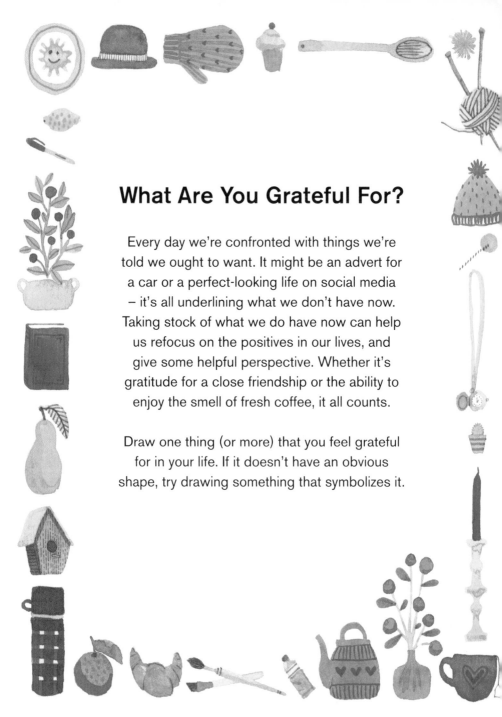

What Are You Grateful For?

Every day we're confronted with things we're told we ought to want. It might be an advert for a car or a perfect-looking life on social media – it's all underlining what we don't have now. Taking stock of what we do have now can help us refocus on the positives in our lives, and give some helpful perspective. Whether it's gratitude for a close friendship or the ability to enjoy the smell of fresh coffee, it all counts.

Draw one thing (or more) that you feel grateful for in your life. If it doesn't have an obvious shape, try drawing something that symbolizes it.

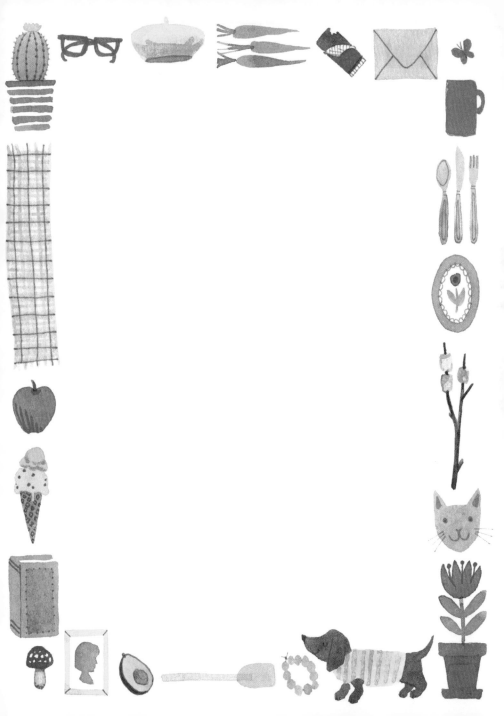

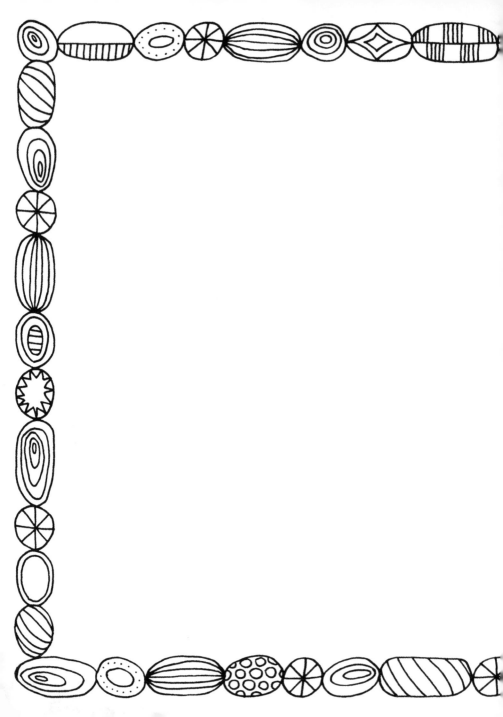

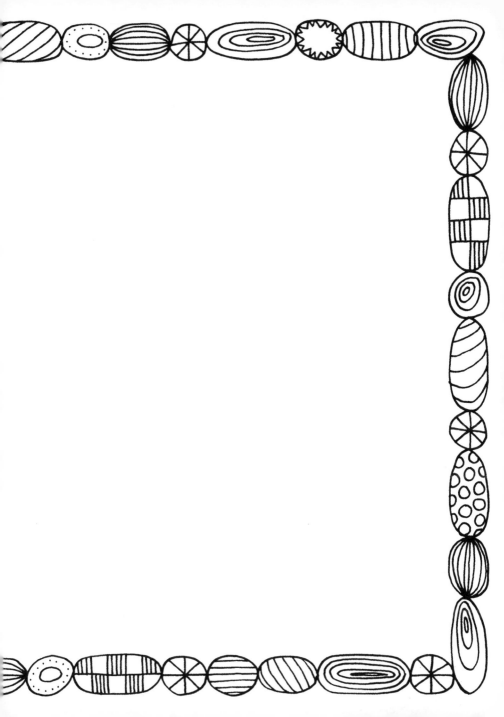

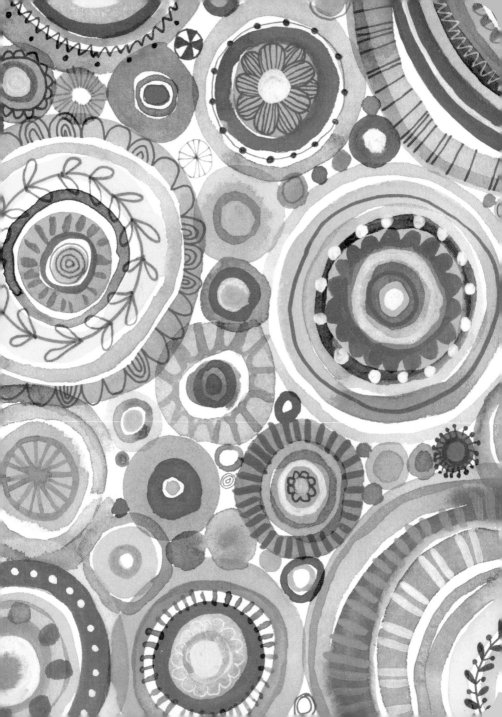

'No one has
ever become poor
by giving.'

Anne Frank

Stress: Identify Your Triggers

Working out what triggers stress can help you anticipate problems and think of ways to solve them. Even if you can't avoid these situations, being prepared makes a difference.

Take some time to reflect on events and feelings that could be contributing to your stress. You could consider:

Issues that come up regularly and that you worry about, for example paying a bill or attending an appointment

•

One-off events that are on your mind a lot, such as moving house or taking an exam

•

Ongoing stressful events, like caring for a family member or having problems at work

Write down your triggers here and start thinking of strategies for how to manage them. It might be as simple as using some of the relaxation techniques in this book.

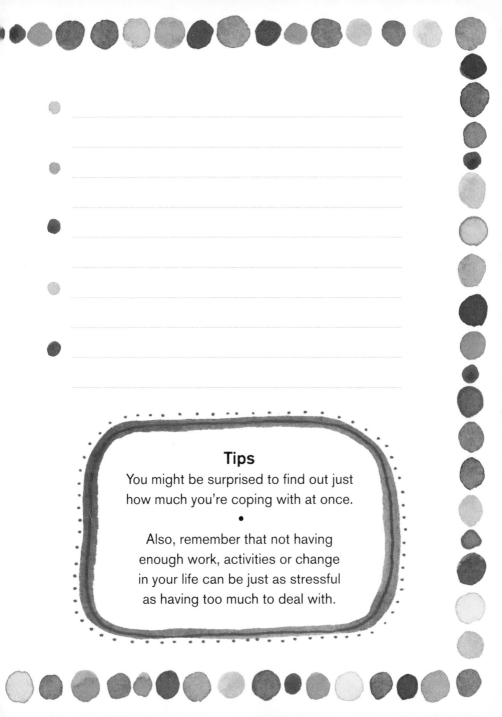

Tips

You might be surprised to find out just
how much you're coping with at once.

•

Also, remember that not having
enough work, activities or change
in your life can be just as stressful
as having too much to deal with.

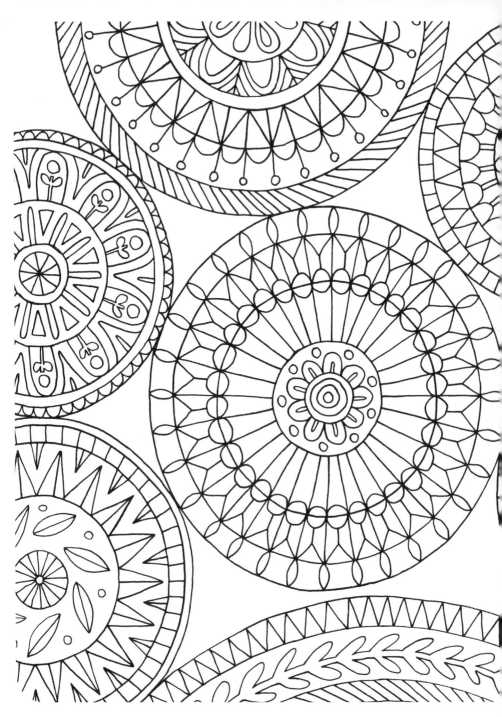

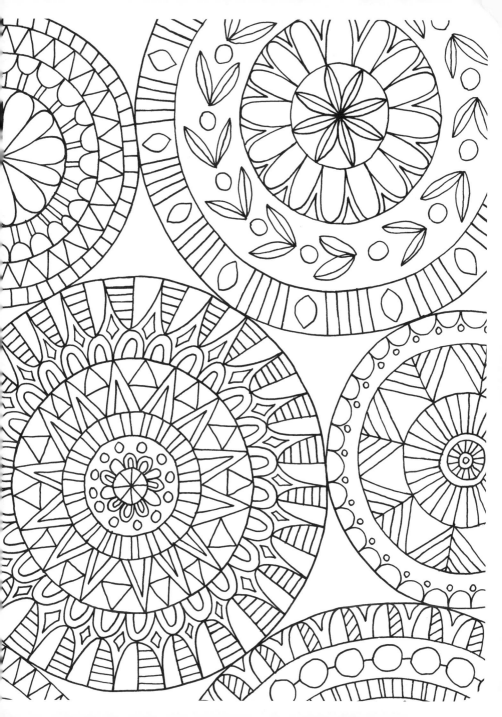

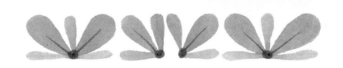

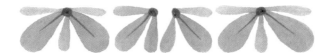

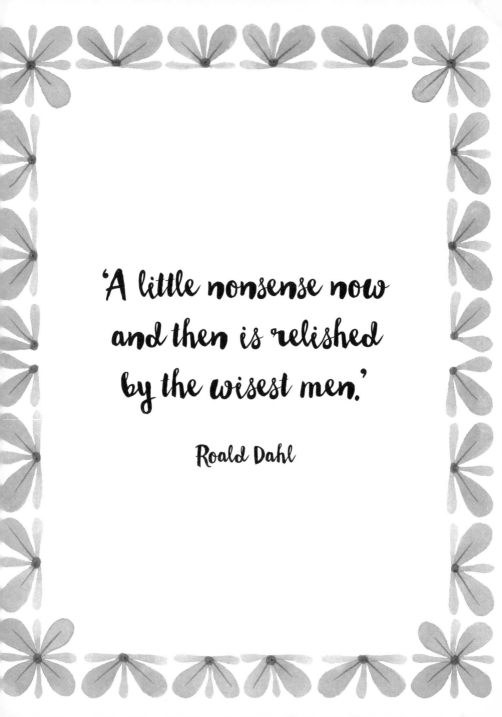

'A little nonsense now
and then is relished
by the wisest men.'

Roald Dahl

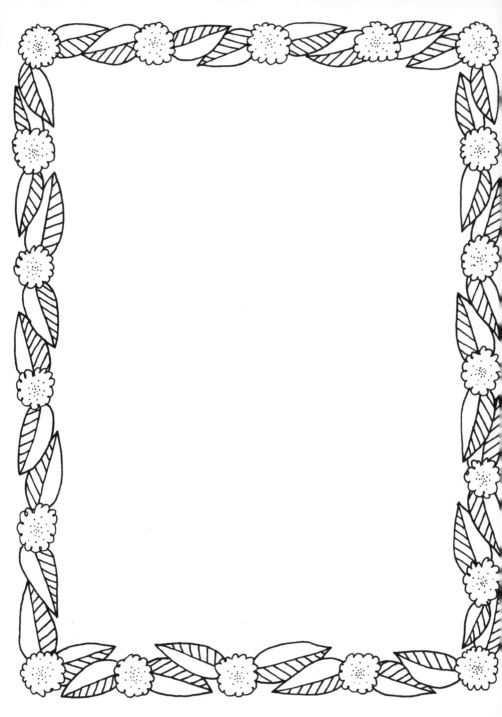

Do a Tech Check

Technology can be great for helping you feel
connected, but if you're using it a lot then it can
contribute to making you feel busy and stressed.
Taking a break, even a short one, can help you relax.

Try turning your phone off for an hour
(or a whole day if you're feeling brave).

•

Step away from the TV, or have an evening where
you don't check emails or social networks. Use
the time to relax doing something else.

•

Identify times when you automatically turn to your
phone, such as when travelling on a train, and plan
to do something else instead like listening to music,
reading a book or doing a bit of colouring or drawing.

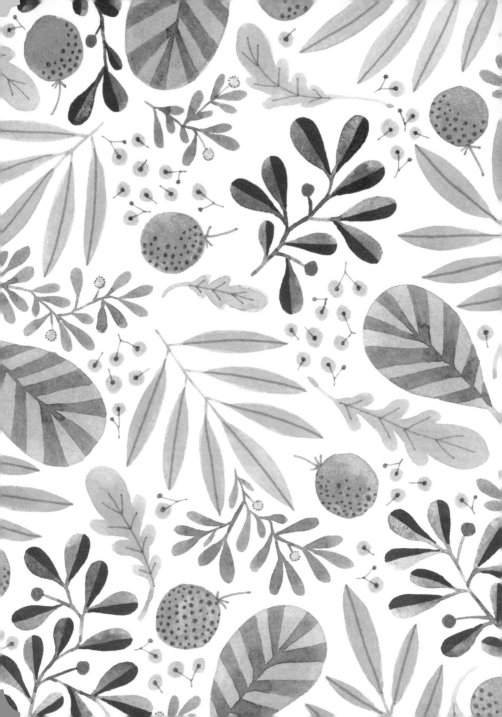

'The moment one gives closer attention to anything, even a blade of grass, it becomes a mysterious, awesome, indescribably magnificent world in itself.'

Henry Miller

Take a Mindful Walk

Spending time in green spaces can reduce stress, anxiety and depression, and gentle exercise is a good way of relaxing. Try this mindful exercise when you're next out on a walk to make the most of what nature has to offer.

1. Find a green space. When you get there, stop for a moment and take a deep breath.

2. Start walking slowly – try not to worry about getting somewhere quickly.

3. Really focus on each step you take. Notice which part of your foot touches the ground first, and feel the transfer of weight through your foot.

4. Think about the rest of your body – how are you holding your arms?

5. Notice the ground underneath your feet. Is it grass or earth? Does the ground feel soft?

6. Listen to the sounds around you – can you hear birdsong, or wind rustling through the leaves?

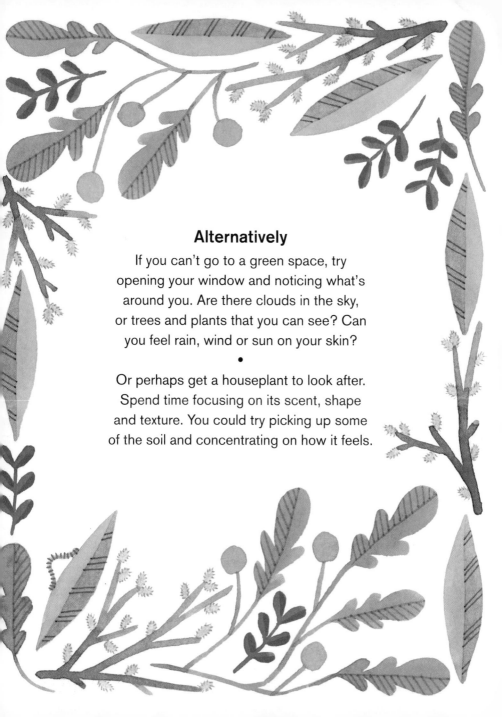

Alternatively

If you can't go to a green space, try opening your window and noticing what's around you. Are there clouds in the sky, or trees and plants that you can see? Can you feel rain, wind or sun on your skin?

•

Or perhaps get a houseplant to look after. Spend time focusing on its scent, shape and texture. You could try picking up some of the soil and concentrating on how it feels.

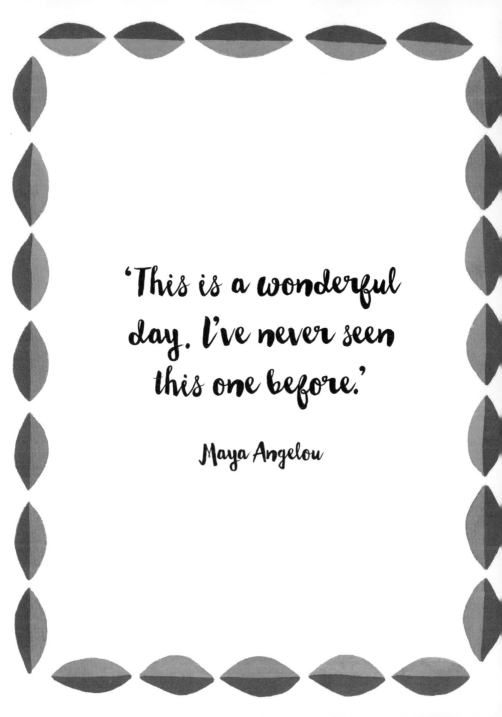

'This is a wonderful day. I've never seen this one before.'

Maya Angelou

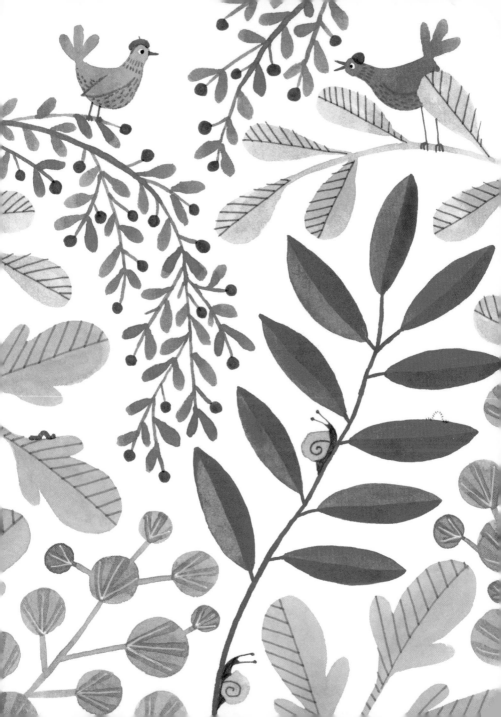

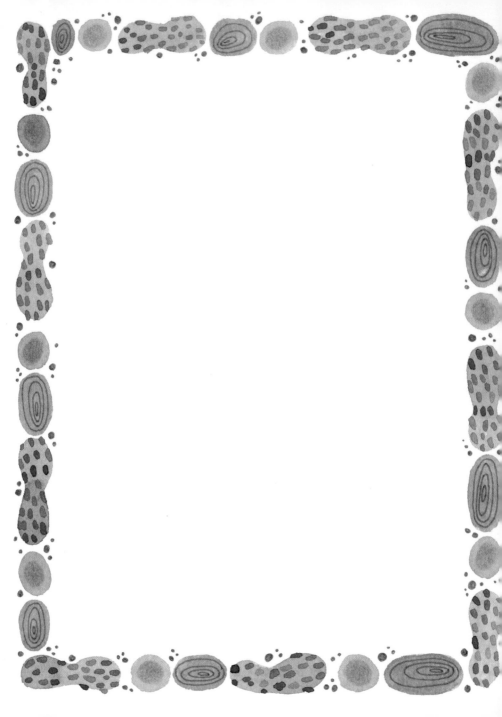

Serene and Tranquil

This is a useful relaxation technique for when you can't easily move about or pick up a pen. For this exercise, all you need is your imagination. Close your eyes if you can, then let your mind transport you to somewhere you feel calm.

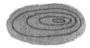

Think of somewhere relaxing and peaceful. You might choose a memory of somewhere you've been or a place you have imagined.

Think about the details of this place. What does it look like? What kind of colours and shapes can you see? Can you hear any sounds? Is it warm or cool? Let your mind drift and your body relax.

Later on, you could draw the scene here.

'If you hear a voice
within you say you
cannot paint, then
by all means paint
and that voice will
be silenced.'

Vincent van Gogh

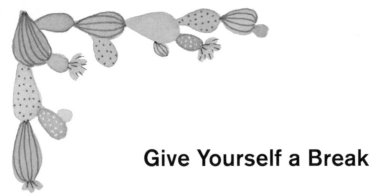

Give Yourself a Break

Learning to be kinder to yourself in general
can help you control the amount of pressure
you feel in different situations.

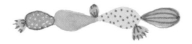

Reward yourself for achievements – even small things
like finishing a piece of work or making a decision.
You could take a walk, read a book, treat yourself to
your favourite food, or simply tell yourself 'well done'.

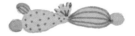

When you're feeling low, look back at the list you
wrote for 'What Do You Enjoy?' and make a plan to
do at least one of those things in the next few days.

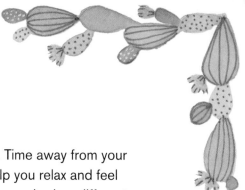

Take a break or holiday. Time away from your normal routine can help you relax and feel refreshed. Even spending a day in a different place can make it easier for you to cope.

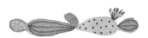

Resolve conflicts, if you can. Although this can sometimes be hard, speaking to a manager, colleague or family member about problems in your relationship with them can help you find ways to move forward.

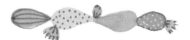

Forgive yourself when you make a mistake, or don't achieve something you hoped for. Try to remember that nobody's perfect, and putting extra pressure on yourself doesn't help.

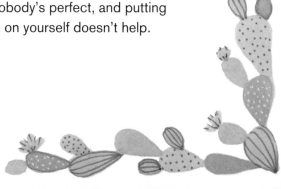

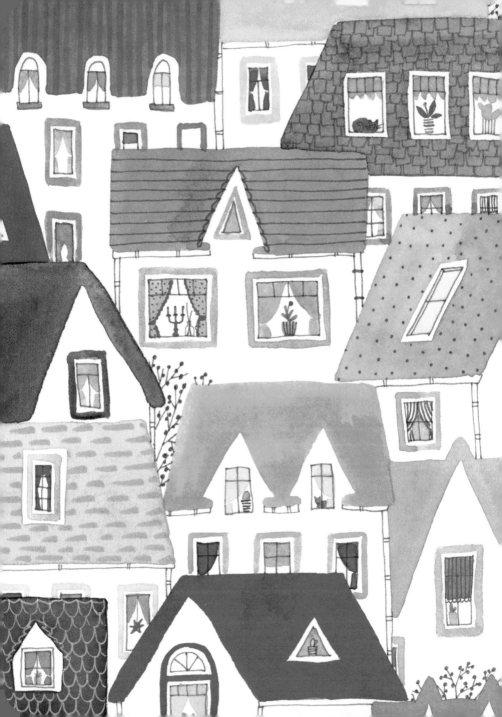

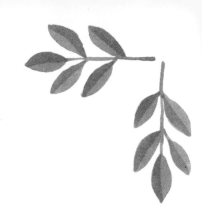

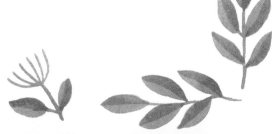

Just Breathe

Learning to breathe more deeply can be an easy way of boosting your wellbeing. This is a really simple exercise and works brilliantly for when you're in the midst of a difficult day and need a moment to collect yourself.

Breathe in through your nose and out through your mouth. Try to keep your shoulders down and relaxed, and place your hand on your stomach – it should rise as you breathe in and fall as you breathe out.

•

Count as you breathe – start by counting to four as you breathe in, four as you breathe out, then work out what's comfortable for you.

•

If you've got a bit more time, you could move on to colouring the pattern opposite while keeping your breathing steady.

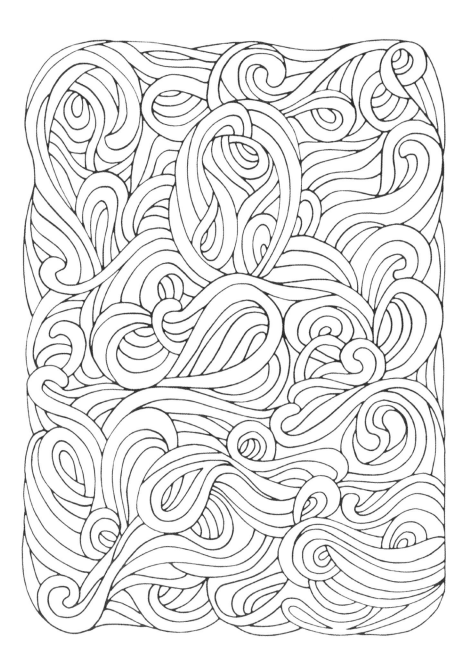

'Whenever your mind becomes scattered, use your breath as the means to take hold of your mind again.'

Thích Nhất Hạnh

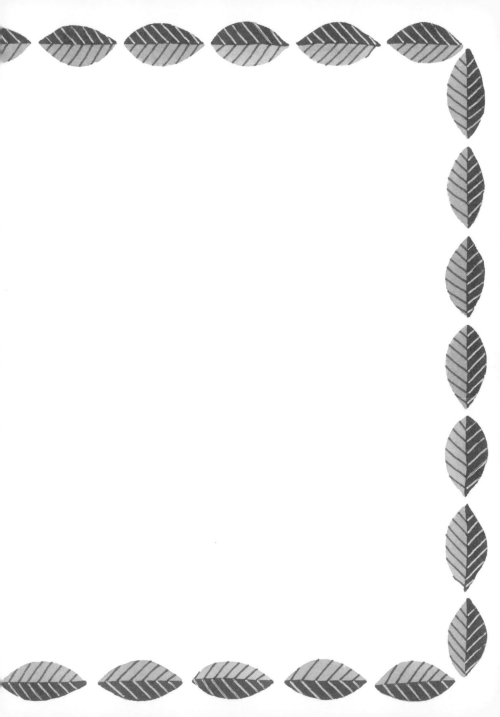

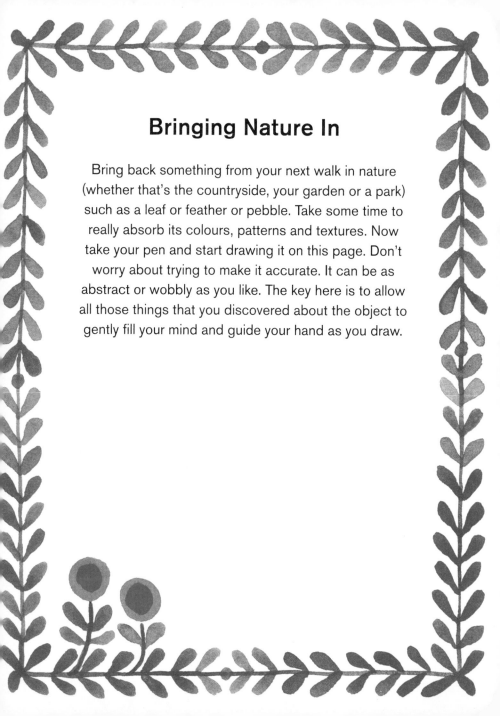

Bringing Nature In

Bring back something from your next walk in nature (whether that's the countryside, your garden or a park) such as a leaf or feather or pebble. Take some time to really absorb its colours, patterns and textures. Now take your pen and start drawing it on this page. Don't worry about trying to make it accurate. It can be as abstract or wobbly as you like. The key here is to allow all those things that you discovered about the object to gently fill your mind and guide your hand as you draw.

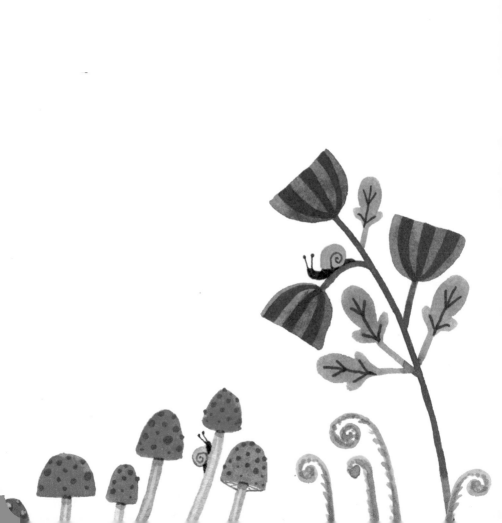